# Take Care, Son

ROBINSON

This edition published in the UK in 2014 by Robinson,
an imprint of Constable & Robinson Ltd

Reprinted in 2016 by Robinson

3 5 7 9 10 8 6 4 2

A CIP catalogue record for this book
is available from the British Library.

ISBN: 978-1-4721-1556-0

Printed and bound in China

Robinson
An imprint of
Little, Brown Book Group
Carmelite House
50 Victoria Embankment
London EC4Y 0DZ

An Hachette UK Company
www.hachette.co.uk

www.littlebrown.co.uk

# Take Care, Son

## The Story of my Dad and his Dementia

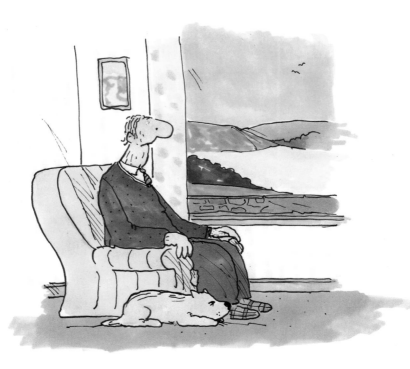

# Tony Husband

ROBINSON

*Hi Dad ... can we have a chat about your dementia ...*
*Can you remember how it started?*

Dementia?

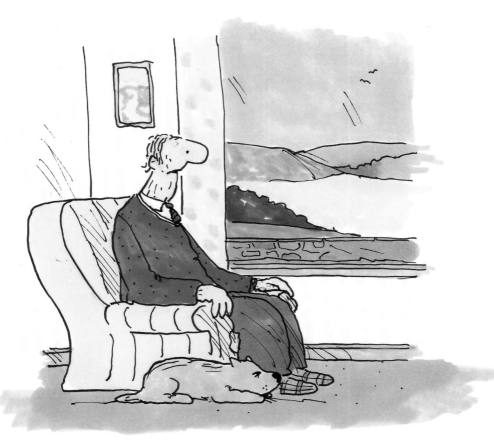

Dementia, is that what I had . . . Ha ha . . . I had dementia and you ask if I remember how it started . . . Ha, that's funny.

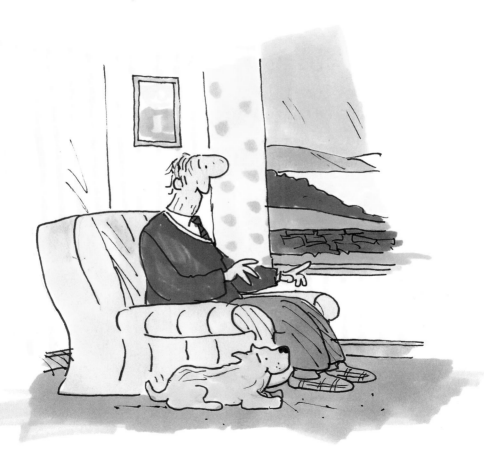

Let me think . . . I mean, it's not like it just starts like a cough or a toothache, it's something that creeps up on you.

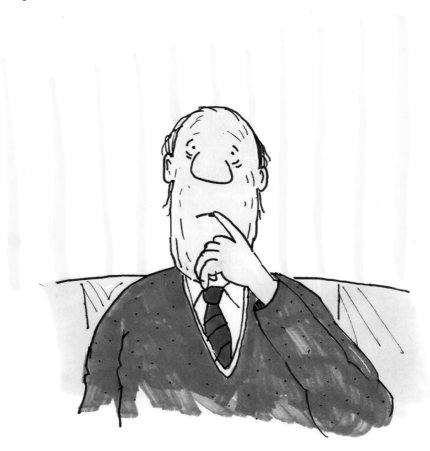

Because when your mum died . . . I threw myself into things . . . I was very active in mind and body. I wasn't going to sink under . . .

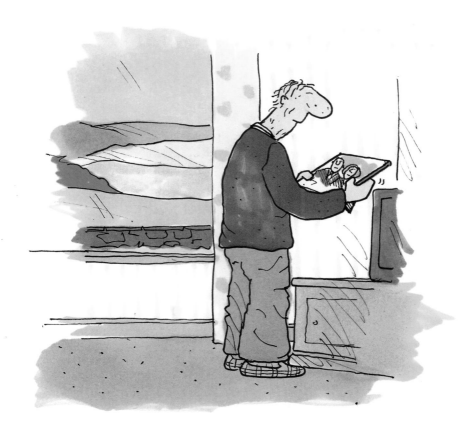

I loved painting . . . watercolours . . . I did my own Christmas card every year. People looked forward to them, you know. Course, I had my pets in every one. Tee hee.

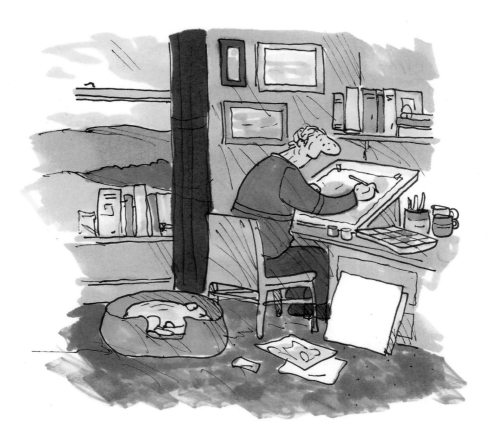

I loved golf . . . I wasn't very good, mind. I did enjoy the company, though, and the exercise . . . and I was the Seniors President too.

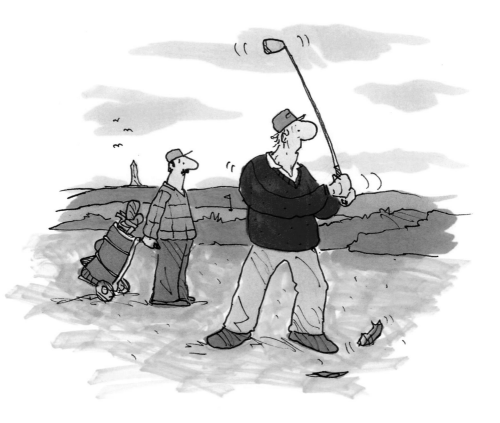

"Fore!"

I liked being involved in the community. I was a bit of a committee man: the golf club; Probis; the War Memorial Trust. I liked a debate, a bit of a fight if I'm honest.

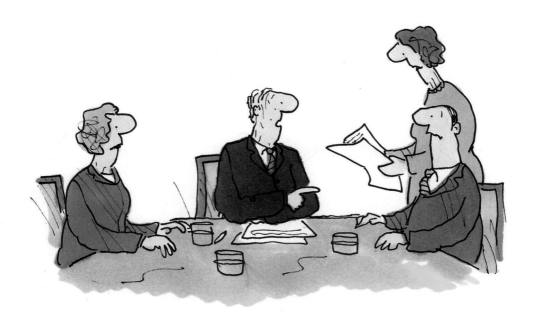

*How about your great achievement? You know, your First World War project.*

Aye? Oh yes, that was an achievement, wasn't it . . . You mean researching all the lads from the town who died in the Great War. Great task, more like . . . phew . . .

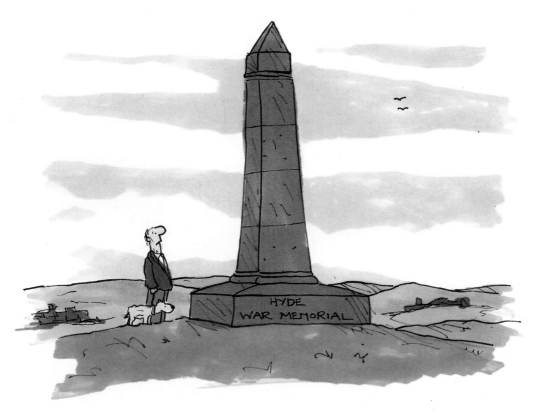

*But Dad, the mental strength it took to do all that research. The hours of research, late nights . . . You were relentless.*

Yes I know! It was hard, but someone had to do it. Someone had to chronicle all those lads who perished. Every single name is now in remembrance books, and I got the council to create a memorial garden. Proud of that, you know.

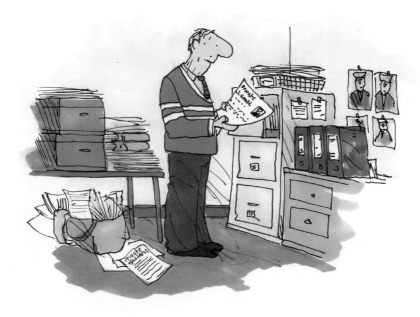

*We were proud of you too.*

I loved playing my piano . . . Boogie Woogie and blues.
. . . I played in bands in the army, I was that good.

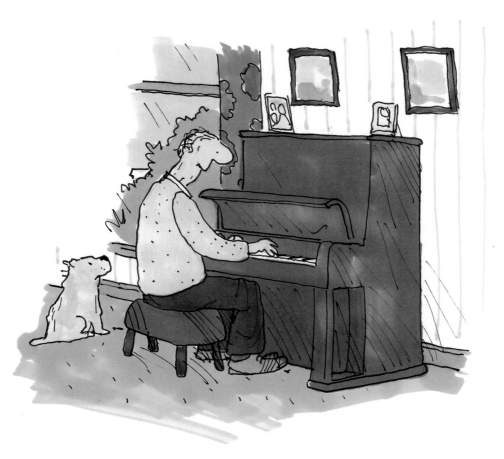

I enjoyed a pint . . . especially with my lads talking football, politics, music . . . you can't beat a pint and a chat in a good pub.

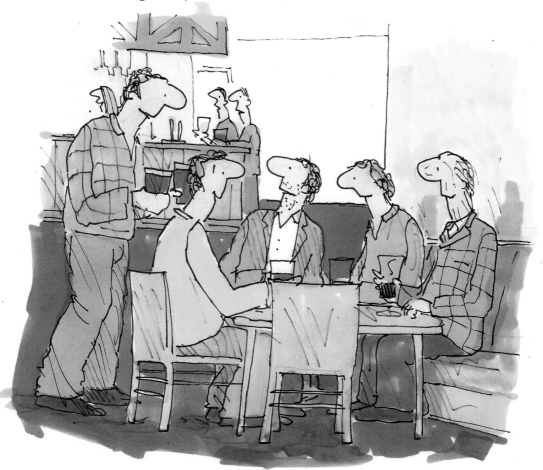

And of course my dog Lossie . . . my lovely best pal.
Always there for me. Kept loneliness at the door.
Oh Lossie.

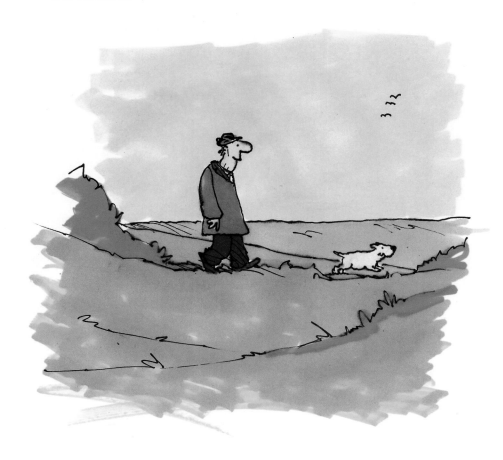

But things began to change didn't they . . . we noticed
you weren't the same but we couldn't pin it down. It
was just a . . . feeling we had.

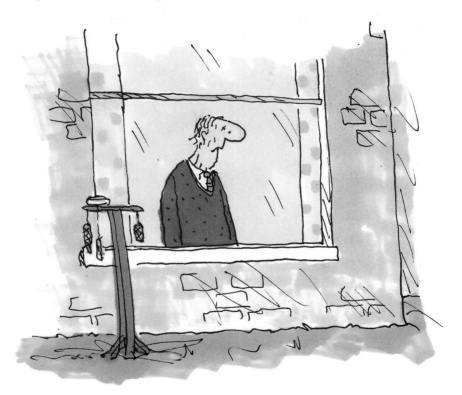

Yes . . . things did change slowly . . . I mean we all
forget, and that's the problem – when do you realise
it's a different form of forgetting?

*So how did it start for you Dad?*

Just that, forgetting things, I suppose. Dates, names,
appointments . . . daft things, important things.

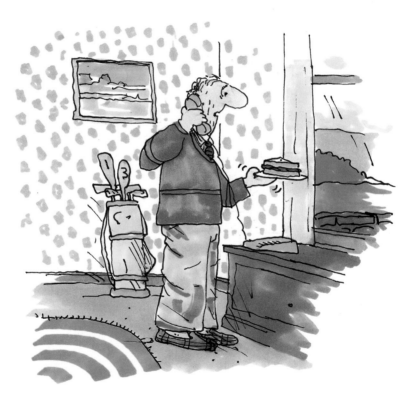

"What, I'm on the tee in ten minutes? . . . bloody hell,
no, of course I'd not forget. I'm on my way."

I'd go out and leave the door open or I'd lock myself out.

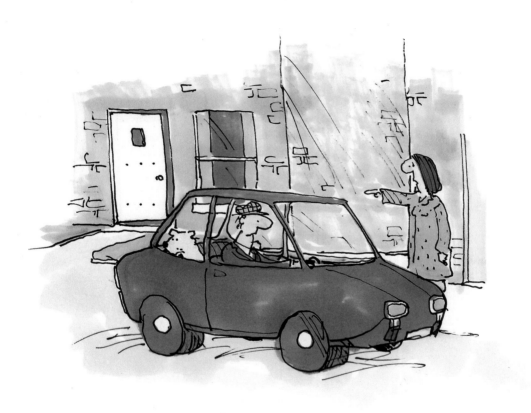

"Ron, your door!"

I left the tap running a number of times . . . flooded
myself out, apparently.

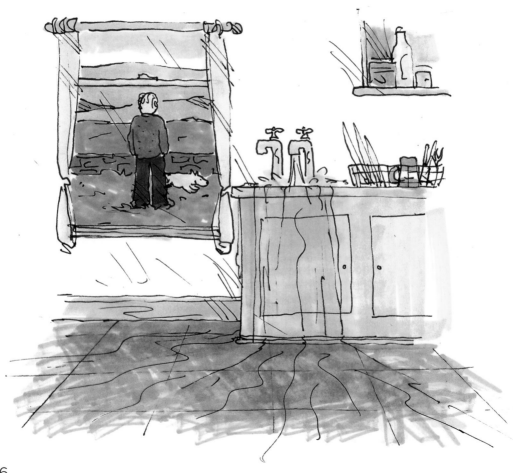

It could be embarrassing.

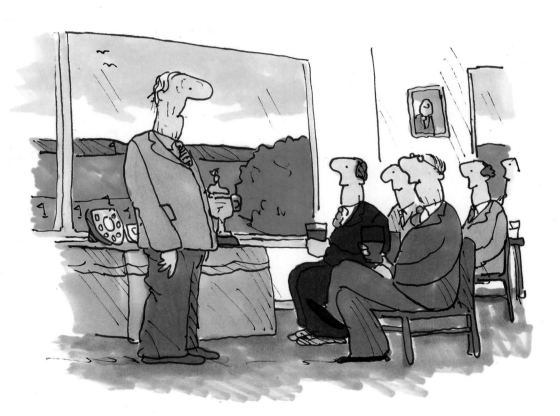

"And the winner of the monthly medal is . . . er . . ."
"Bloody hell, Ron, it's you! Ha ha."

And going out in my pyjama bottoms wasn't the wisest move.

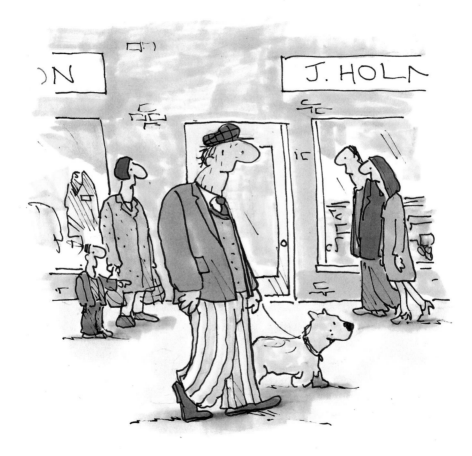

The strange thing was, though . . . my distant memory
cleared up. I could remember stories I'd long forgot
about my childhood.

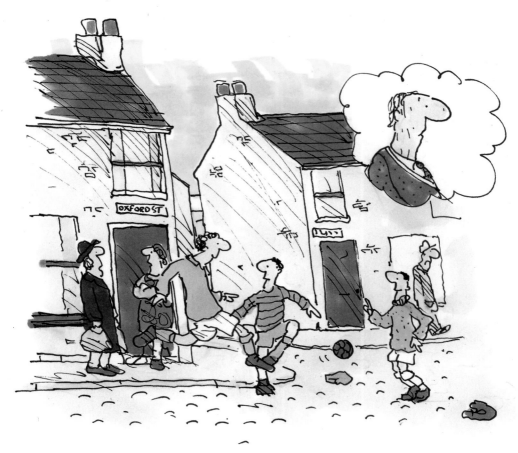

And my wartime experiences . . .

*Yes, you told us some, er . . . interesting stories.*

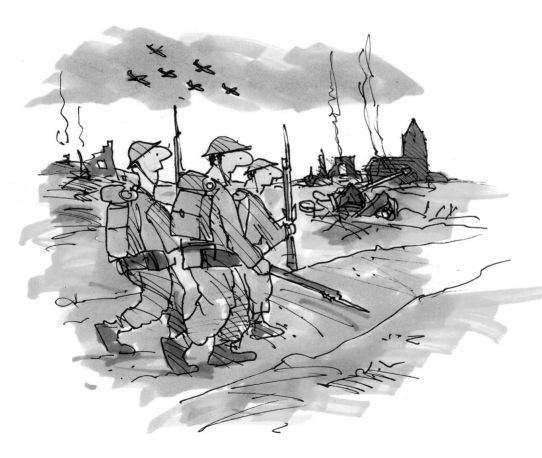

*Do you remember the anxiety?*

Yes . . . I didn't like the post. It scared me, letters from people I didn't know. They all wanted money, the doctors, tax man . . . One said I owed them £25,000!

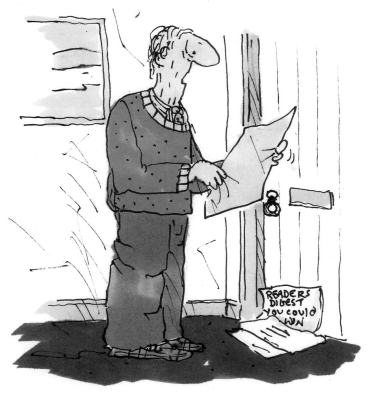

*It was actually a note from* Reader's Digest *to say that you were in the £25,000 draw. You didn't win by the way.*

And I didn't trust anyone, not even my family . . .

*Er . . . especially your family.*

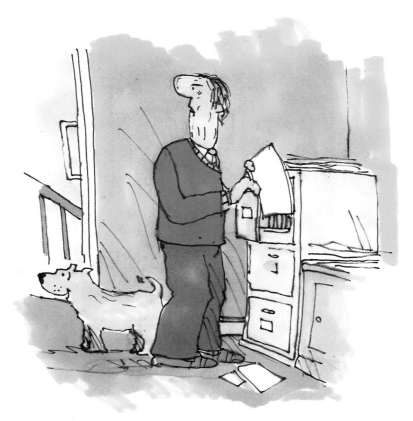

"Hi . . . it's us."
"Come to get my money, I bet. Well, you're
not having it."

*Do you remember the ghost?*

There was one I'm sure . . . I felt its presence often. I'd put things down, like my wallet on the window ledge, and then it would vanish. I'd find it days later in the fridge or somewhere. It was very strange.

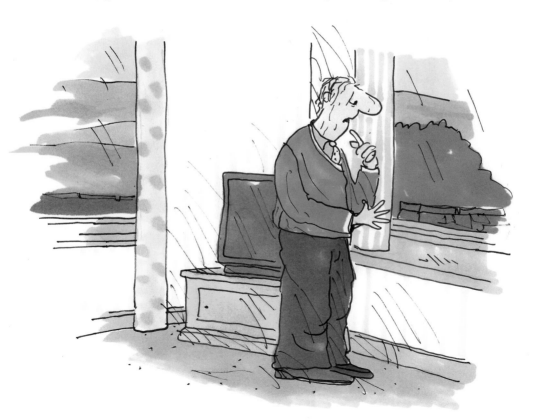

*That's when we all decided to take you to the doctor . . . we were getting worried.*

I didn't want to go . . . got annoyed about it. All those questions, how was I supposed to remember all that? Ridiculous!

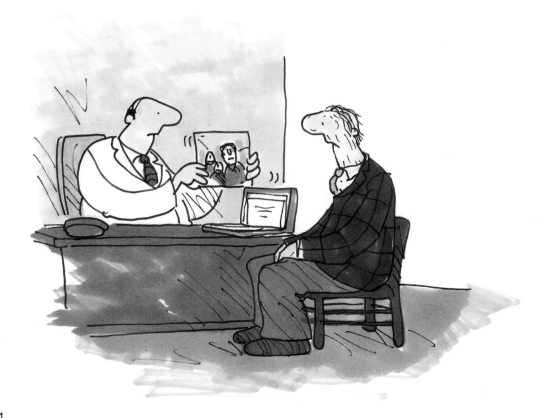

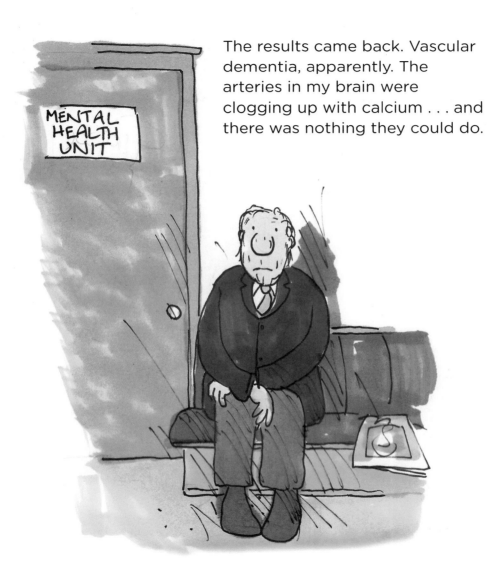

The results came back. Vascular dementia, apparently. The arteries in my brain were clogging up with calcium . . . and there was nothing they could do.

And if hearing that wasn't bad enough, I had my car taken off me. That was hard to take. My independence was being eroded bit by bit. I felt isolated, lost . . .

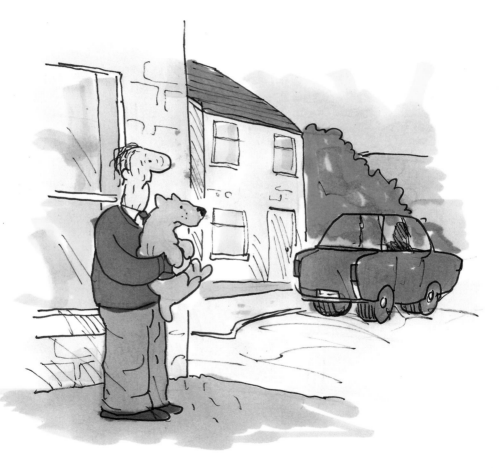

*We had no choice, Dad. You were a liability on the roads.*

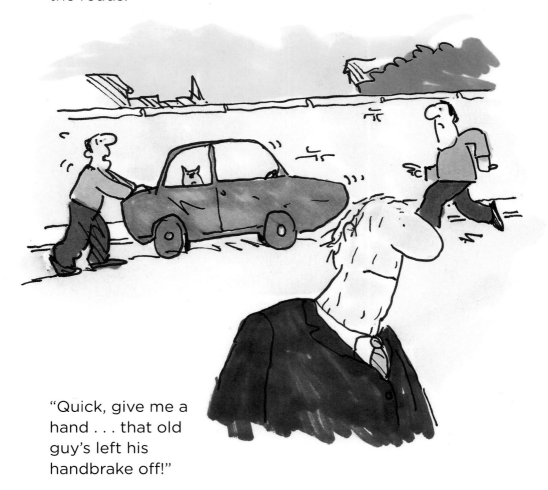

"Quick, give me a hand . . . that old guy's left his handbrake off!"

*We contacted social services who, it must be said, were very good. They asked what you needed, took note of what you needed, too.*

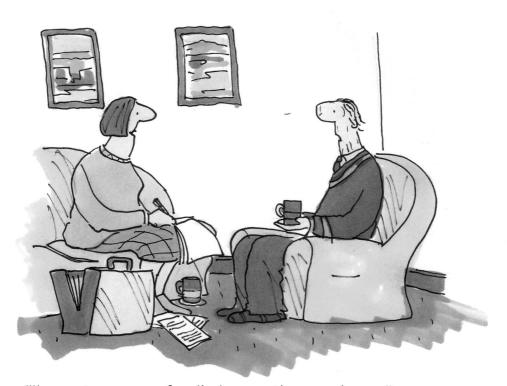

"I've not seen my family in months, you know."
"They're in the back room . . . they've been
  with you all day, love."

Yes, and the carers got involved . . . They were fantastic, I loved their visits, so friendly and chatty.

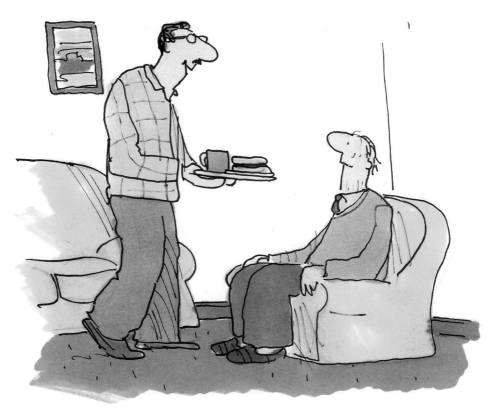

"I'll just tidy up, then sit and have a chin wag. Here's lunch for now."

But when they went . . . I felt lost, lonely. It was like everyone had stopped calling. I wondered where you all were.

*Oh, I remember the phone calls, 40 or 50 a day, the same questions . . . Bloody hell.*

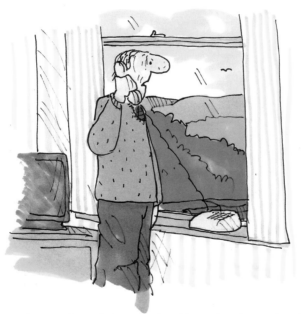

"Hello . . . have I got to go to the doctors today?"
"We went this morning . . . I'm trying to work here, Dad. . ."

*Then we'd feel guilty for being annoyed with you.*

Do you remember the aliens, ha ha . . . I thought there were aliens flashing messages to me, so I sent them messages with my blinds in Morse code,

Turned out they were car headlights on the road across the valley . . . dearie me.

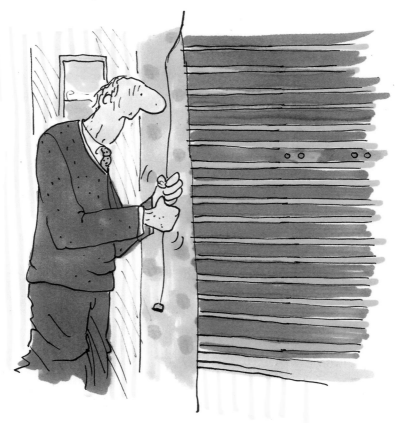

There were people coming to my house all the time too. I didn't know half of them. Were they carers? Were they forgotten friends? They all seemed nice, and it was company.

"Lovely paintings, mate. Worth a few quid, aye."

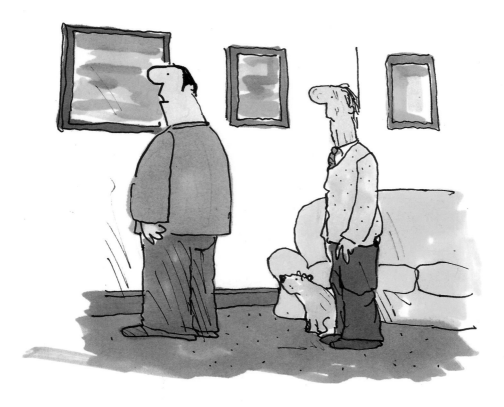

*Yes Dad, that worried us. We knew people were calling in . . . and they weren't all carers. And you couldn't remember who they were.*

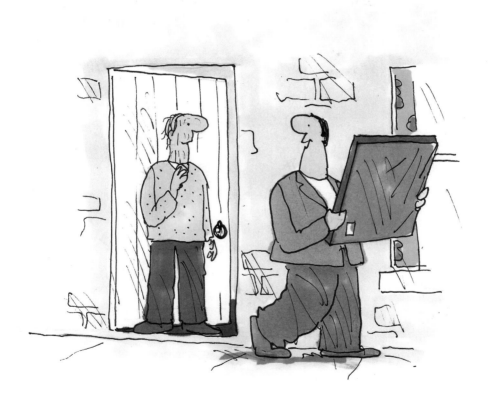

"OK mate . . . I'll take this painting and get it valued for you."

I remember a fire, I think . . . was there a fire?

*Yes . . . you left a chip pan on . . . a lot of smoke, but not much damage and no one hurt. But it was a big warning.*

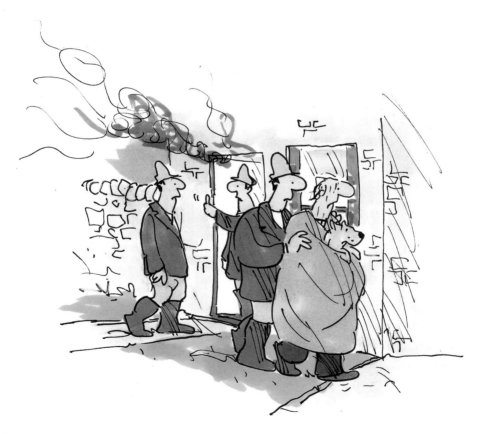

*We knew then we needed more help, you needed more care. We went to see the doctor.*

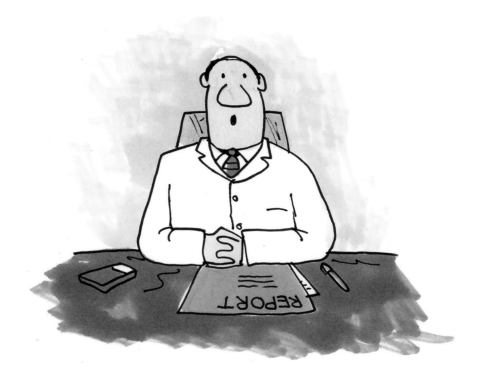

"I think the time has come for your dad to have 24/7 care . . . you need to start looking for a suitable placement for him . . . I'm sorry."

Leaving my home was heartbreaking. But I couldn't remember at the time why it was . . . I just knew that something had gone for ever.

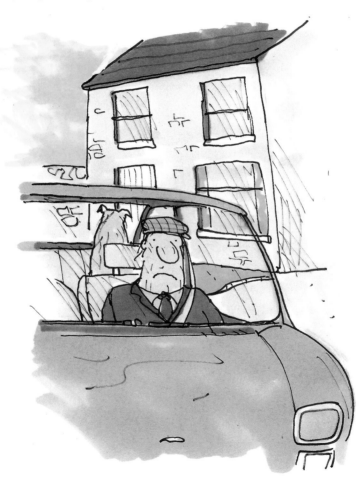

And then I couldn't have my dog . . . They took Lossie off me.

*The dog was fine, Dad. He was with us and he came to visit, you remember . . .*

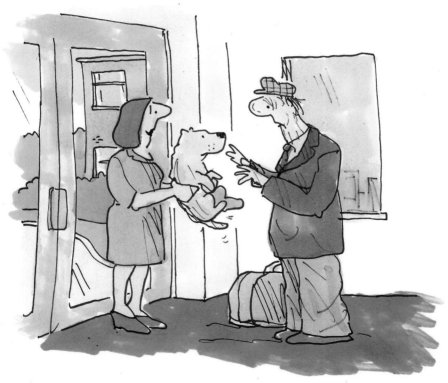

"He'll come and see you soon."

The care home was nice though, very warm. I had my own room and television, though I didn't know how to turn it on. There was a picture of me outside my door, so I'd know it was my room.

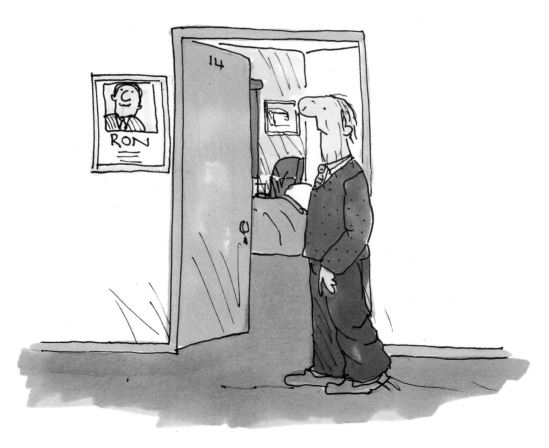

I had a garden to go into, but the door was always locked. I had lots of photos of everyone . . . but with all that, I still missed something. And I didn't know what it was.

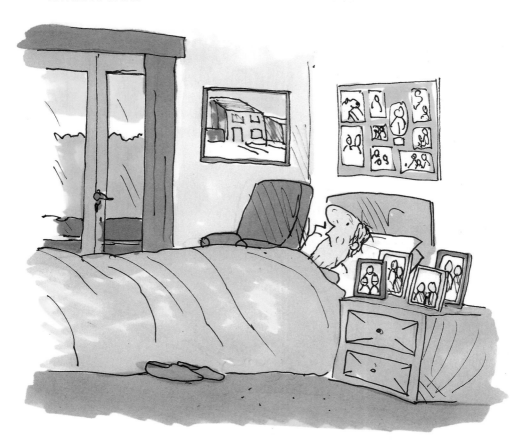

But for us – your family – it was such a relief to know you were safe and being looked after. You had full-time carers . . . we could visit when we wanted.

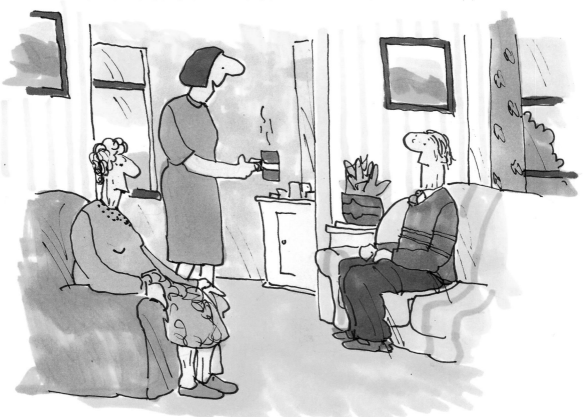

"Tea up, everyone. "

And I had company . . . Oh yes, and I had a girlfriend too . . . I remember.

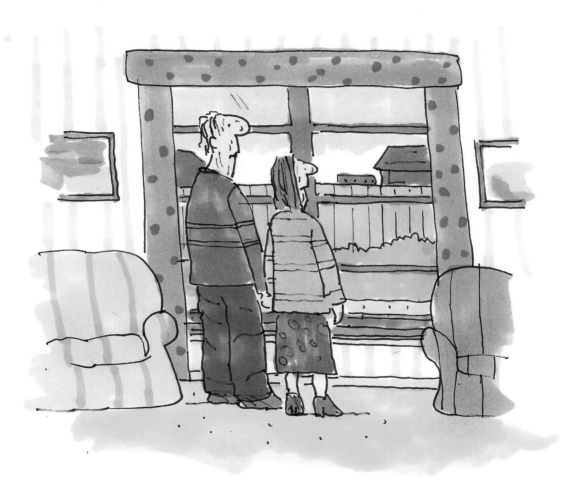

We went everywhere together . . .

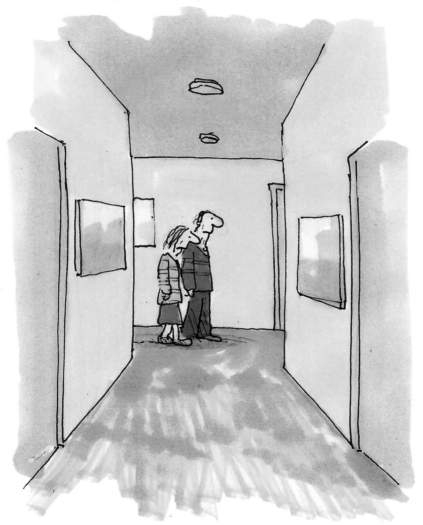

*Tell you what, though. There were some characters in there . . .*

You can say that again, off their trolleys most of them. Ha!

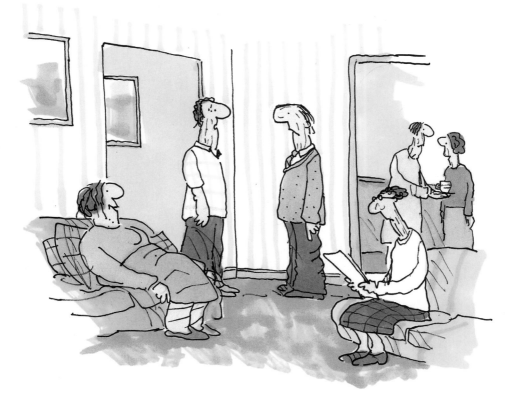

"Eee you're handsome . . . are you married?"
"Have you got any spoons? Why did I just ask for spoons?"

At least we weren't miserable like that lot in the geriatric part of the home. They just sat staring at the TV, saying nothing to anyone . . . depressing.

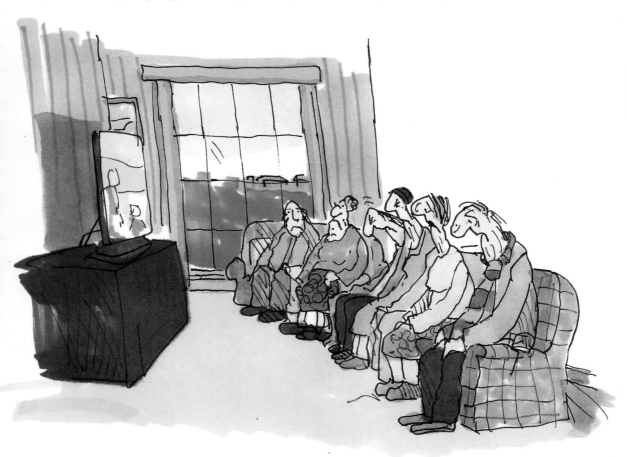

And when Lossie came to visit, it cheered everyone up . . . She made us smile.

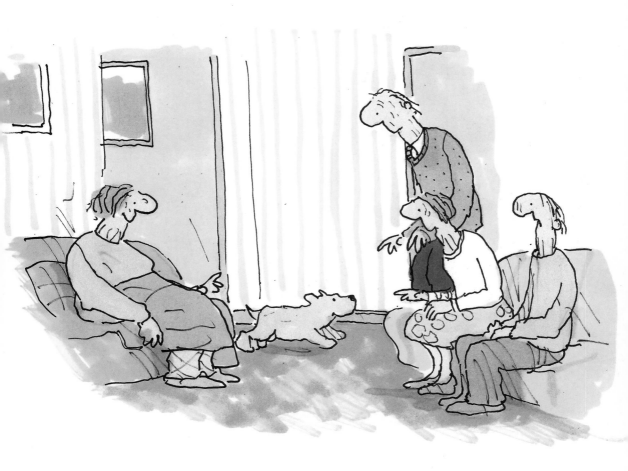

Course, I had my music still . . . Do you know, it never left me. Never left any of us really. We'd have dances and sing-songs and play piano and we had lovely times.

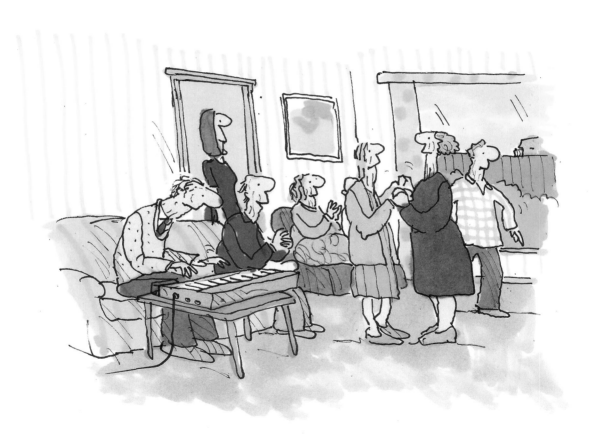

*We realised the one thing that stayed was your music.*
*Word for word, note for note . . . it never left you.*

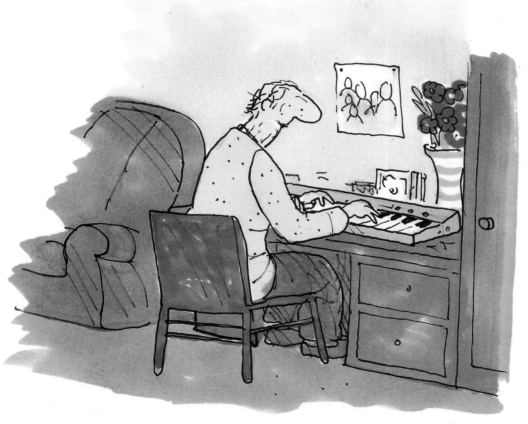

Yes, music gave me freedom.

*I remember you came for Christmas dinner that last time. We were playing Low's Christmas album. They do a wonderful version of 'Silent Night'. You hadn't said a word all day, but as the song started you put your knife and fork down and sang along with them. It was beautiful and moving . . . it was like a memory had just clicked. When the song stopped you picked up your utensils and started to eat again in silence.*

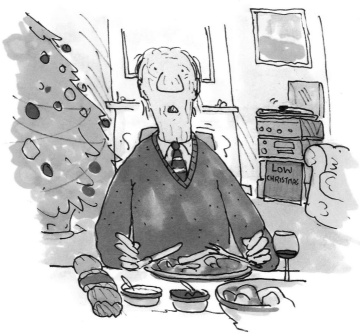

"Silent Night . . . holy night . . . all is calm . . . "

I liked it when one of you took me out. It was a change. Sometimes I thought deep down I was going home. Sometimes, though, I wanted to get back as soon as possible. I felt anxious outside that home . . . everything was overwhelming, frightening.

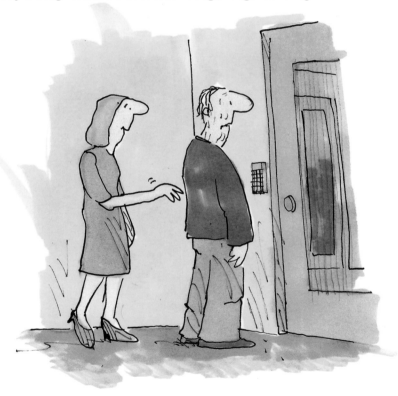

"Come on back Ron, we'll make you a cuppa."

My memories were confused, jumbled . . . nothing made sense, the world I knew was disappearing, it didn't make sense and I presume I didn't either.

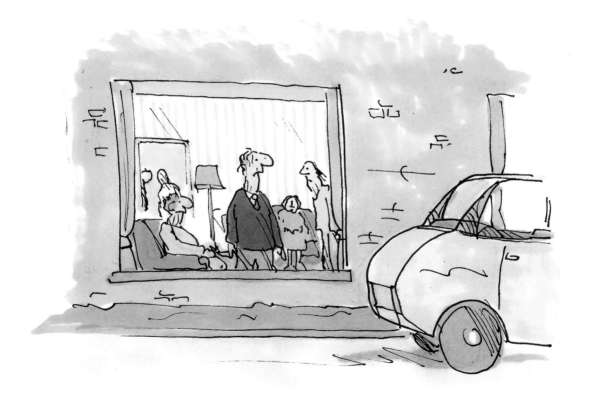

*Yes, we knew things were deteriorating now . . .*

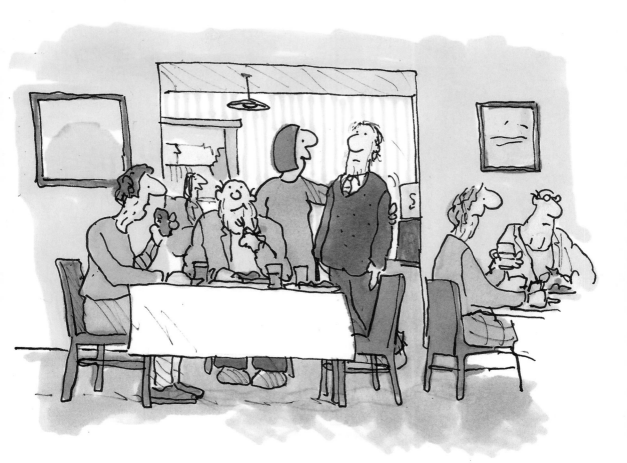

"Come on Ron . . . have some dinner . . ."

*You rarely left your bed, you didn't recognize any of us, you
even stopped playing your music. Our only comfort was that
you were protected, warm . . .*

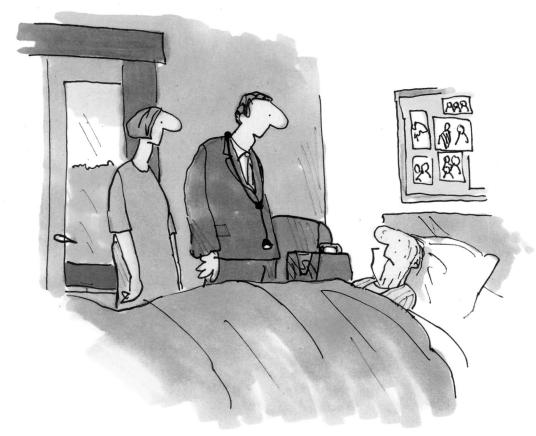

"Hello, not getting up again . . . let's have a look at you then."

I just wanted to stay in my room . . . My world was shrinking, my mind was shutting down . . .

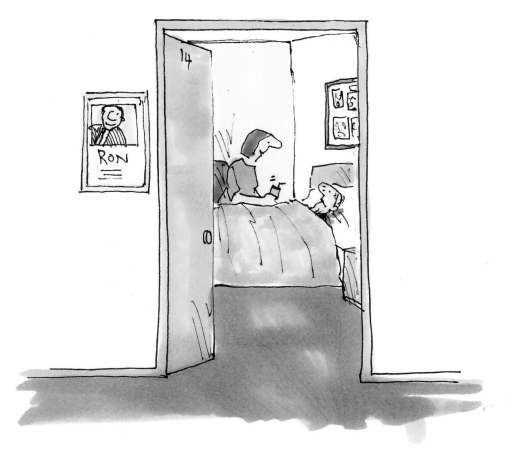

"Ron, try one more drink . . ."

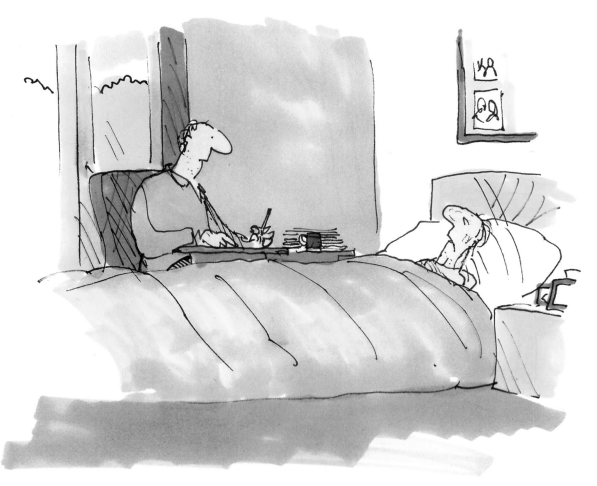

*I remember one time, though. I'd spent a few hours with you in your room. You slept, I worked. Then, when I left and said goodbye, you replied, clear as a bell . . . "Take care son." It took me aback. They were the last words I heard you say.*

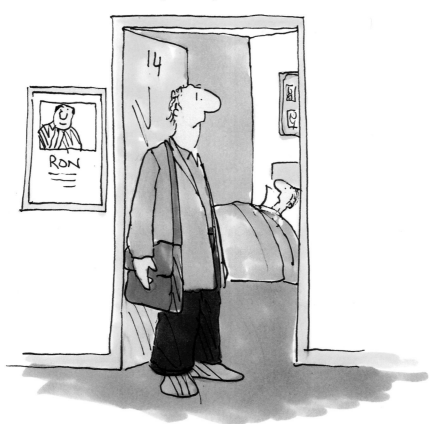

*It was like a candle flickering back to life for a moment . . . then it went out for ever.*

It was all very scary. Imagine a day when nothing will mean anything to you.

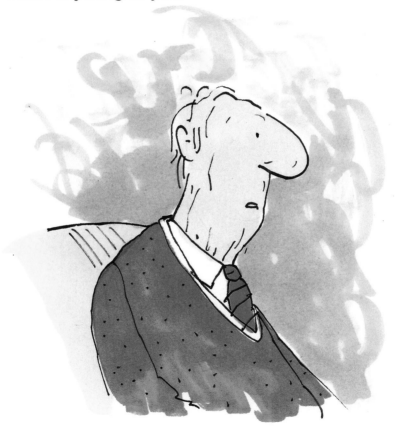

Every memory of everything and everyone you loved and cherished would be wiped away . . .

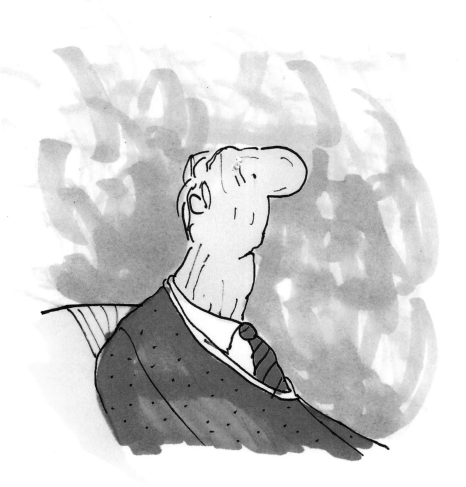

When you love life as I did and you loved your life as I did . . . can anything be so cruel?

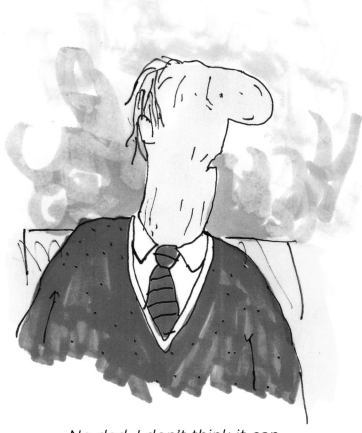

*No dad, I don't think it can.*

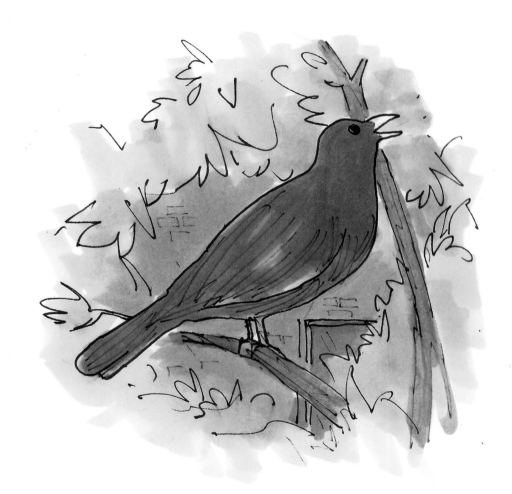

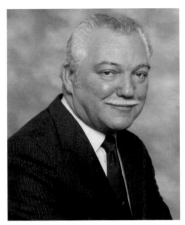

Ron Husband, 1925–2011

If you are concerned about yourself, or about someone you know who may have difficulties with memory or the ability to do everyday activities, it is important to talk to your GP.

If you, or someone you know has dementia, it may help to know you can get support and talk to somebody as and when you need to. There are national organisations who may have local services for the person with dementia and their family members/carers, and who can provide you with practical, emotional and signposting support.

These are just some of the dementia helplines in the UK.

| | |
|---|---|
| Admiral Nurse Direct Helpline (part of Dementia UK): | 0845 257 9406 |
| Alzheimer Scotland: | 0808 808 3000 |
| Alzheimer's Society Helpline: | 0300 222 1122 |
| Northern Ireland Alzheimer's Helpline: | 028 9066 4100 |
| Wales Dementia Helpline: | 0808 808 2235 |
| Dementia Web Helpline: | 0845 120 4048 |
| Moodswings Helpline: | 0161 832 3736 |
| Life Story Network | 0151 237 2669 |

It is important to know that Alzheimer's is just one form of dementia (there are over a hundred different types of dementia) and any of these helplines will be able to offer you support regardless of the type of dementia.